WILLPOWER

*How to Achieve your Goals by
Making a Plan and Sticking to
it with Self-Control, Discipline,
and Ease*

by **K.B. Bryson**

TABLE OF CONTENTS

INTRODUCTION

Life, as complicated as it may be, is the offspring of the choices, decisions, and actions that we make and take on a daily basis. From trivial things like deciding on the color of your tie, to mind-boggling choices you may make over the course of your career, your decisions and actions will add up to have significant impact on the course of your life. One of the mysterious, and often elusive, things that attributes to these day-to-day life choices and actions is "Willpower."

People often blame the lack of their own willpower as one of the key barriers to change. According to a recent survey by the American Psychology Association, nearly 3 in 10 Americans cite the lack of willpower as one of the key hurdles in achieving their own life goals. The inability to discipline and control one's self often results in faulty choices and poor decisions. Goal-setting may be a good starting point in working towards your plans but if you cannot sustain it with the right amount of discipline and willpower, then achieving those goals will certainly be an extra difficult task.

Most of the world's famous leaders exhibit willpower. They learn and acquire new skills, cope with daily challenges, and achieve short- and long-term goals using self-discipline and willpower. Is willpower something that can be learned? Or is willpower simply inborn? What can you do to control the amount of Willpower you have? This book will address these questions in order to provide a comprehensive guide in having the willpower to so that you will be more able to set and achieve goals.

CHAPTER 1 - WHAT IS WILLPOWER?

According to the Merriam-Webster dictionary, willpower is "the ability to control one's self." It enables an individual to accomplish a task despite its difficulties. In a nutshell, willpower is your inner strength that guides you in taking action, making a decision, and doing a task despite any complexities. Willpower is what separates human beings from animals. The ability to accomplish a task amidst a delicate and complex situation using an organized thought pattern gives us the luxury of being on top of the food chain.

It enables us to establish our motivations, distinguish rewards from punishment, and have full control over our mind and body. For example, a person with a strict dietary plan is bound to meet a lot of temptations. The enigmatic gap between goal-setting and accomplishment is where willpower plays in action. Will you stick to your diet, or give in to the temptation of binge eating? Will you come up with an excuse to exceed your calorie limit, or will you fight your cravings? The answers to these questions will determine the course of your goals which are greatly attached to your self-discipline and willpower.

Hence, willpower or self-control *is* something that you can learn and improve, at any point in your life, should you choose to do so. You can even replenish willpower for every task carried out. By increasing and replenishing your

Willpower, you will actually be enabled to adapt to all kinds of challenges, and resist temptations.

CHAPTER 2 - DISCOVERING THE PSYCHOLOGICAL ASPECTS OF WILLPOWER

There is solid academic research discussing the foundation of willpower and its association with our everyday life. If you think willpower is just some vague word concocted to falsely raise your hopes, you are wrong. Willpower, when utilized to its maximum potential, can lead to bigger things that could beautifully alter the course of your life.

In psychology, willpower is defined as the person's ability to avoid short-term temptations in exchange for long-term goals. It is characterized as the drive, determination, and self-control to achieve a plan.

For psychologists, the ability to inhibit our impulses, feelings, and compulsion enables us to gain control over our decisions. This self-control separates us from animals because we can clearly distinguish urges and set out ways how to curb them. This is associated with the activity and size of the brain's frontal lobes. Human beings have larger frontal lobes indicating our capacity to think, decide, and plan rationally. Our ability to control sexual urges and impulses, for example, enables us to work well within a group, accommodate other human beings, adjust to the needs and requirements of the situation, and work smoothly in a balanced ecosystem.

Some studies also suggest that the level of glucose in our body has an effect on our ability to self-control. People who want to quit smoking can lengthen their resistance against the urge to puff on a cigarette when their level of glucose is increased. That is the reason why many people attempting to quit smoking may resort to energy drinks containing glucose.

Willpower gets exhausted, too. You need to replenish it, especially when using it quite often. It's a limited amount of energy that should be used wisely. This is why you may find it difficult to go to the gym after a long hard day at work: all the stressful events you experienced during your work day may have actually exhausted your willpower for that day.

CHAPTER 3 - DEVELOPING WILLPOWER AND DISCIPLINE

Many people say that one's destiny is not based on pure chance, but instead it is based on solid choices. "Life is what you make it," as the popular adage goes. The previous chapters have explained the concept of willpower and what it means in your life. Hence, it can be said that having willpower is one of the main ingredients in achieving your life goals. So how do you develop willpower and self-discipline? Where do you get your motivation? How do you accomplish your goals?

Let me explain the road to willpower and success into the following steps.

How to Develop Willpower

Find your Focus

We live in a world where people and things are in constant need for attention. From the constant hustle and bustle on our streets, to our constantly ringing cell phones and incoming text messages, it is no wonder that our attention span is shrinking day by day. If you want to work your way towards success, then it is imperative that you find your focus. So, how do you do that? Limit all your distractions in life one by one, until you can eliminate them altogether. For example, if you're spending hours each night on FaceBook, why not trim that down to a half hour per day? Set an alarm to time yourself.

Do this until you can totally eliminate useless hours on social media sites, or limit it to twice a week for half hour each time. The key is not to ignore the distractions but to get accustomed to a situation where the object of distraction is absent, or you are in control over it. You can also up the ante by applying this limit-eliminate rule on other bigger personal distractions, such as your cell phone. You don't need to keep it with you everywhere you go, at all times. Remember back in the days before cell phones existed? We got along just fine going out into the world on a daily basis and only checking our messages when we returned home in the evening. Start slow, by putting your cell phone in a drawer with the ringer off for an hour or two while you prepare and eat dinner. Then check it afterwards, just one time, and put it away again until the next morning. Slowly but surely, you can wean yourself from this dependency of a distracting device.

What are your biggest distractions? And what will your plan be to tone them down?

Know your Weakness

The ability to be fully aware of your weaknesses gives you a venue for improvement. Once you have embraced your flaws, you will have a clearer picture of how to improve them. For example, if procrastination hinders you to accomplish tasks, the first step to improving this is by being aware that you suffer from procrastination. Once you have accepted this fact, it will be easier for you to work on eliminating the problem. On the other hand, people who are often in denial of their weaknesses tend to get stuck in one stage. Keep in mind that our life is divided into different phases. It is normal for one person to be sad and unmotivated—this could just be a phase. But once that person does not do anything to get out of that phase, he becomes stuck—and being stuck at one phase is the biggest hindrance to moving forward with your life. That is why it is very important for you to identify your weaknesses before you can start working on improving them.

So, what are your weaknesses? Write them down now. Seeing them in ink on paper will make them more real and undeniable.

Start with Small Tasks and Decisions

You can move on to bigger decisions once you become comfortable making these willpower changes with smaller tasks first. Starting with small tasks enables you to gain skills and experiences that will shape your future decision-making abilities. In other words, your experience in handling small tasks will prepare you for bigger and more complicated puzzles in life.

What are some small things in your life you'd like to change as "practice" for the bigger ones? What bigger changes are you trying to make, that you will start to focus on as soon as you get the hang of changing the smaller things?

Learn to say NO

Are you the type of person who always tries hard to please people? If yes, you are in the danger zone. Being a 'yes' person all the time is not only tiring, but also cowardly. It also says a lot about your inability to get your message across. Hence, it is very important that you know how to refuse— politely. Saying 'no' without being rude may vary from one situation to another. If you are faced with a really pushy person, try saying "I'm sorry, I don't think I can make it." This short and polite statement is the universal translation of "no." If someone is inviting you to do something but you can't because you have other commitments, you can say "I'm sorry I can't make it but I can..." and then mention your interest in other opportunities in the future. You also have to keep an eye on giving false hope. If you think that you really can't make it, then it's better to tell the person early on instead of keeping their hopes high for nothing. Avoid using the word "maybe" or "perhaps."

When did you recently say "yes" or "maybe" when you really wanted to say "no"? How should you have responded in that situation instead?

Reward yourself

Recognize yourself each time you accomplish something no matter how small it is. Psychologists have actually cited the presence of reward as one of the key sources of motivation. Give yourself a pat on the back whenever you ace an exam or close a deal. You can also bank on material rewards to inspire you more to work harder. Rewards should not be misconstrued as bribes for yourself to make something happen. Instead, rewards should be taken as your motivational tools to get you where you want to be faster. Later, in the following chapters, you will learn the psychological explanation behind the concept of reinforcement/reward and the role it plays in getting work done.

What reward(s) can you think of that would be motivational for you? Write down a few things that you could "give" yourself as a reward if you were to accomplish something great?

Keep in mind that the answers to these aforementioned questions are just the starting point to accomplishing your goals. Being able to actually act on your motivations and apply your skills are the next step in making your goals a reality.

How to Stick to your Plan

Creating a goal, a plan, or a rule is one thing, but actually sticking to it with all your heart is another. While the aforementioned steps on how to improve your willpower will help you in attaining your goal, if you do not stick to them on a regular basis, then you would have to start all over again each time you are faced with a task. That is why being

20

consistent with your goals is very important. So how do you do it? Here are some simple ways:

Be Specific

Vague plans often get ignored because you don't know exactly where to start. It's not enough to say "I want to be happy." You have to define what happiness is and what will make happy. Happiness is such a vague concept that varies from person to person. This means to say that one's happiness is not synonymous to the rest of the world's definition of happiness. This also applies to smaller scale decisions and life goals. For example, if you want to reduce your weight, then set a time frame for yourself. Always know when you're starting, and when you're supposed to finish. Your timeframe will condition your body and mind to get used to a routine.

Monitor your Progress

Keeping an eye on your progress is very crucial so that you will have a clearer picture of what has been accomplished and what is still needed to be done. Achieving a goal is very much like going for a long drive. You check on your distance travelled against the estimated time of arrival so that you get a clearer picture whether or not you are close to your destination, and you prepare yourself mentally for the remaining portion. If you need to have an actual progress tracker to help you, then so be it.

If this is what it takes to keep you focused and specific in achieving your goal, then do it. There are some online apps you can download on your phone which help track progress. If you're not the techie type, then go back to basics. Draw a simple chart on a piece of paper, and write down your specific goal, time frame, and track your weekly and monthly progress there.

Learn to Rise Amidst Failures

Failures are inevitable. If you have the right mind set, you can even use failures to your advantage. Learn from your mistakes and know how to rise above them. Keep in mind that when a journey starts and things do not go as planned, it is always okay to start from the beginning. That is the ecosystem of life. Knowing how to handle failures and being aware that failures are inevitable will actually help you stay committed to your plans and routines in life.

Write Down your List of Motivations

Ask yourself, the following questions:

"Why am I doing this?"

"Who am I doing this for?"

"What will I get from this?"

Once you have clear-cut answers to these questions, write them down. This list will be your constant reminder that you are on your journey towards achieving your goal, and you have some darn good reasons to do so. If you are more creative, get a piece of cardboard and collage onto it some cut-out pictures from magazines that symbolize your motivation. Do you want to have a sexy body? Add a picture of your favorite model, and a picture of your favorite vacation destination where you plan to be in your bikini looking gorgeous next year. Are you saving up for something in the future? Cut out a picture of your dream car or dream house. You can even include quotations that will inspire you to persevere and work harder. Every time you lose track, don't get upset with yourself, but instead just return to these visions that motivate you, and this will help you get back on track in no time.

CHAPTER 4 - OVERCOMING THE HURDLES

The road to achieving your goals won't be complete without encountering a few hurdles. Keep in mind, these hurdles will actually make your victory that much sweeter. The key challenge is learning how to face these hurdles while staying committed to your plans.

How to Resist Temptations

If Adam and Eve didn't bite the apple, then the story of our lives would probably not be the same. Indeed, temptation is such a tough thing to handle, whether or not you look at it from a religious perspective. Your road to achieving your goals is likely to be tainted with temptations. Some are lucky to have the stamina to refuse these, but for many, the task of saying "No" to temptation is an uphill battle.

Take the case of someone who is trying to lose weight as an example. There are many temptations lurking around the corner throughout the weight loss process. The person may be tempted to binge eat or exceed the require amount of calories, or simply join his or her coworkers in enjoying a slice of cake when celebrating the boss's birthday at work. This is why it's important that you go through this process step by step. You're not trying to lose all your weight in one day by starving yourself, and you don't have to skip having that piece of cake altogether (unless you want to). You're in this for the long haul, and in the grand scheme of things, although all of these little choices add up, none of them make it or break it alone. So if you're just starting off on your diet and trying to build up your willpower little by little, try this: Accept the piece of cake, but concentrate on eating only half of it instead of the whole slice. Let yourself truly enjoy the half you eat, but then immediately toss the other half in the trash can. By starting off with small (doable) changes, such as eating half of the slice, instead of the whole thing, you have neither deprived yourself, nor have you fallen into the black hole of temptation. Just know, that as you become healthier and healthier over time, you will eventually reach a point where you wouldn't even want the cake! Yes, it's true!!! This time next year, the thought of cake will seem gross to you. But don't force that on yourself too early, or else the cake will become the juiciest of forbidden fruit, and the temptation will only rise.

You can also resist temptation by using physical space, and just stay away from the actual location of the temptation. If you think you are going to break your commitment by going to the Boss's Birthday party, then wish him a happy birthday that morning, and find schedule something else during his party that will keep you away. Don't put yourself in a situation where you know temptations could arise and you're not ready or willing to handle them. Simply being absent in a situation of potential temptation is a strong action in and of itself. This way, you've killed two birds with one stone:

avoiding temptations, and sparing yourself from decision-making and possible guilt.

Overcome Decision Fatigue

Your willpower functions just the way your body muscles do. Thus, when used over and over again, your willpower can also suffer from fatigue. Coined by some psychology experts as "decision fatigue," this phenomenon is a struggle for those people who are constantly faced with the task to decide. Think of judges in court. There's a controversial study that says judges in court who suffer from decision fatigue are likely to say no to parole requests. Like court judges, you are also very prone to decision fatigue. Under this condition, the brain starts to get tired of making a decision so the default answer to every situation becomes a no. In effect, you might even make very poor decisions that do not take into consideration the pros and cons of every situation. If your assignment at work requires heavy decision-making, then you are likely to feel drained at the end of the day. You might be better off opting for certain de-stressing or rejuvenating activities (i.e. hitting the gym) but what happens instead is your brain may go easy on itself by resorting to the default decision (i.e. just stay at home) which does not require much thinking. If this sounds familiar, then you are probably suffering from decision fatigue.

Decision fatigue, which refers to the deterioration of your decisions, is normal and can be dealt with. But once it starts to trample on your big-time decisions, then decision fatigue becomes a roadblock to success. So how do you overcome this? First, start making commitments instead of mere decisions. For example, before your long hard word day even begins, write down in your calendar "6pm Spin Class at the Gym". This way, when 5:30pm rolls around, you don't even have to exhaust your brain by forcing it to make a decision. The decision was made when you wrote it down in your calendar. Now all you have to do is drive over to the gym, without thinking at all. This type of advanced and specific commitment making is a terrific tool in preventing decision fatigue from ruining your goals.

You can also overcome decision fatigue by focusing on your priorities. Sure, there are tons of things to decide upon, but you can't accomplish them all at the same time. So, using your list of priorities, do the most important thing first before jumping into the smaller ones. This will enable you determine and appreciate the things that matter to you the most. Invest your energy and effort in acting on tasks that have the biggest and most positive impact in your life.

CHAPTER 5 - REWARDING YOURSELF

Chapter 3 briefly mentioned the importance of rewards in gaining willpower and accomplishing a task. There's a popular experiment worthy to be mentioned now. In the 1960s, psychologist Walter Mischel conducted his "marshmallow experiment" among 1000 kids. In the experiment, kids were asked if they want a marshmallow now or if they want to wait for two marshmallows in 15 minutes. As the lives of the same children were followed for years to come, Mischel discovered that the kids who waited the 15 minutes for the two marshmallows (high delayers) became more successful (academic- and career-wise) later on in their lives. There were also lower rates of marital divorce among those who waited. In essence, the study suggests that people who know how to delay gratification will achieve bigger things in the end.

While the thought of a sumptuous dessert may be really tempting, the thought of a sexy body is more alluring, once you fight the urge to give up on your diet. When we were young, we were trained in an environment where for every good deed, there's a reward waiting for us. For example, in order to motivate us to get good grades in school, our parents would promise us material things such as toys and candy. These situations have conditioned us to study harder in an attempt to ace the exams in order for us to get the rewards. Of course, as we move on to the next phases of our lives, challenges become more complicated as rewards become more attractive.

In achieving your goal, it is important to fix your eyes on the long-term goal instead of the short-term temptations. Rewards, when set properly, can get you to work and motivate yourself to move on to bigger heights. Recognizing your achievements may be done in a graceful and strategic manner that won't make you look like you are bragging about your accomplishments.

First, know how to schedule your rewards. Why not indulge in your favorite meal after beating a deadline? Or treat yourself to a full body massage after your successful presentation? Of course, the weight of your rewards gets heavier as the tasks grow more complex. Long-term goals require delayed gratification. For example, if you are planning to save up on your car, then you might have to give up your monthly shopping spree. This is where indulgence limitation comes into play. You need to moderate your cravings, wants, and desires in order for you to achieve a long-term goal. Last, know when to take a break. Doing an enormous task can take a toll on your emotional and physical abilities if you do not take a break. It will only drain your brain which could result to poor decision-making process. So, it is very important that you set small breaks while accomplishing a task.

CONCLUSION

Willpower is a very important aspect in our life. It is our bridge to transitions and personal growth. Willpower separates us from animals because it enables us to think rationally and act on something using a comprehensive thinking pattern. However, willpower is not something we are born with; rather, it is something that we should all continuously work on as we move on to the next chapters of our life. We should replenish the power of our will in order for us to gain better traction in this world. Like our body's muscles, our brain's ability to decide can also get fatigued. That is why it is important to take breaks and recognize ourselves through rewards whenever we are working our way towards something.

Rewards are also important in conditioning ourselves while doing a task. Delaying gratification is proven to have longer and bigger benefits. While willpower may not be something that you are born with, it can still be developed through time. Willpower can be enhanced by starting with smaller tasks, then moving to bigger ones. It can also be strengthened through constant practice and commitment to your goals. Having willpower is one of the biggest ingredients in achieving your life goals.

Thanks for purchasing this book, and I hope it helped put you on the path to developing and growing your willpower reserve. Willpower is an amazing thing, with incredible power, and we all should be working on strengthening it daily. If you enjoyed this book, please take a moment to submit a review for it on Amazon – I'd really appreciate that!

OTHER RECOMMENDED RESOURCES

Here are some additional resources you may find helpful, especially if your quest for more Willpower is related to wanting a better body and healthier lifestyle.

1) **"Overweight No More: Ten Small Adjustments you can make Today for BIG Weight Loss and a Whole New You"**

   http://www.amazon.com/dp/B00KS4BBEW/

   http://amzn.to/1s5C79V

2) **"Exercise Motivation, Determination, and Discipline: How to Get into a Regular Exercise Routine, Stay Focused, and See Results Fast"**

   http://www.amazon.com/dp/B00LF9I7CI/

   http://amzn.to/1rfsIKe

3) **"How to Stop Sugar Cravings: Discover How to Overcome Sugar Addiction and Stop Sugar Cravings"**

   http://www.amazon.com/dp/B00LKUHOJO/

   http://amzn.to/1kfLMD5

4) **"Increase Metabolism: Start Losing Weight and Burning Body Fat Today with these 25 Effective and Simple Ways to Boost your Metabolism"**

http://www.amazon.com/dp/B00KR0YOSC/

http://amzn.to/SwyM4e

5) **"Self-Confidence: 25 Proven Ways to Boost your Self-Confidence to Overcome Anxiety, Fear, & Self-Doubt"**

http://www.amazon.com/dp/B00LOWOQGC/

http://amzn.to/1kNdkQe

6) **"Lose Weight Easily: How to Lose Weight (Without Weird Diets or Crazy Workout Regimens) for a Healthier Life"**

http://www.amazon.com/dp/B00LQ99TMY/

http://amzn.to/1m2uOrn

Printed in Great Britain
by Amazon.co.uk, Ltd.,
Marston Gate.